Unlocking Quantum Health

Healing Beyond the Natural:

The Quantum Key to Whole-Body Wellness

by

Dr. Robert Rodich

Unlocking Quantum Health

Healing Beyond the Natural:
The Quantum Key to Whole-Body Wellness

by

Dr. Robert Rodich DD., Ph.D.

9436 Impala Drive
Foley, Alabama 36535
USA

www.DocRodich.com

Unlocking Quantum Health

Healing Beyond the Natural: The Quantum Key to Whole-Body Wellness

Copyright © 2025 Dr. Robert Rodich

The views and content expressed in this book are those of the author and may not necessarily reflect the views and doctrine of Dr. Ron Horner or of LifeSpring International Ministries, Inc.

Unless otherwise noted, all scriptures are from the AMPLIFIED® BIBLE, Copyright© 1954, 1958, 1962, 1964, 1965, 1987 by the Lockman Foundation Used by Permission. (www.Lockman.org)

All rights reserved. This book is protected by the copyright laws of the United States of America. This book may not be copied or reprinted for commercial gain or profit. The use of short quotations or occasional page copying for personal or group study is permitted and encouraged. Permission will be granted upon request.

Any trademarks mentioned or used are the property of their respective owners.

Additional copies available at docrodich.com

ISBN 13 TP: 978-1-962808-20-0

ISBN 13 eBook: 978-1-962808-21-7

Cover Design by Darian Horner Design (www.darianhorner.com)

Images: 123rf.com #181866926

First Edition: June 2025

10 9 8 7 6 5 4 3 2 1 0

Printed in the United States of America

Table of Contents

Acknowledgments i

Recommendation iii

Introduction vii

Chapter 1 Quantum Review 1

Chapter 2 The Health of Our Spirit 11

Chapter 3 The Health of the Soul 17

Chapter 4 The Health of the Mind 21

Chapter 5 Doing More Cleanup 25

Chapter 6 More to Think About 35

Chapter 7 The Human Body 39

Chapter 8 Our Emotions 43

Chapter 9 Hormones and More 49

Chapter 10 DNA 51

Chapter 11 My Medallions 55

Chapter 12 Diet, Exercise, and Personal Discipline 59

Chapter 13 Nutritional Testing 67

Chapter 14 Heavenly Engagements
and Heaven's Wellness Clinic 75

Chapter 15 The Blood of Jesus... 79

Chapter 16 Conclusion.. 85

Appendix A 91

Appendix B 93

Gemstones 93

Medallions 97

Description 105

About the Author 107

Acknowledgments

I would like to acknowledge the role that angels and those in the cloud of witnesses play in our earthly assignments. In my own life and in the lives of my children, I have witnessed the hand of angelic intervention numerous times.

One such moment occurred when my son Jason was running across the street to our babysitter's house. A large truck was barreling down the road toward him. I screamed, "Jason!" Just then, he hit an invisible wall with such force that he bounced backward and landed on his rear. At first, I feared he had been struck by the truck. But then I realized—he had collided with something supernatural. The driver of the truck turned ghostly white before my eyes, clearly shaken. And Jason? He was completely unharmed.

Another time, I was working on my car, replacing the universal joint. Lying beneath the vehicle, I knocked the driveshaft loose from where it was attached. Suddenly, the car began to move, threatening to roll right over me. At that moment, I saw the driveshaft lift back into place, holding the car steady just long enough for me to roll out of the way. The instant I was safe, the driveshaft dropped to the ground. I had already dislodged it—there was no natural explanation for how it could have lifted itself back into place. But God!

Then, there is the cloud of witnesses. They are not dead. They have transitioned to Heaven and are as alive as we are. Before my father passed, I made a deal with him—I asked him to ensure that those of us still on earth would receive the revelation and resources we needed to complete our assignments. In other words, my dad became my inside man.

A few months after his passing in late 2019, I received a message from a woman I barely knew. She told me she had seen me in Heaven with my dad at a gathering on a heavenly mountain retreat. She said we had spoken to her, and both of us had expressed our desire to help pastors.

Yes, those in the cloud of witnesses assist us and are likely to be aware of the significant events in our lives. So, to the witnesses and the angels, I offer my deepest gratitude for all that you do.

Recommendation

I am thrilled to recommend this book by Doc Rodich, as well as his voice analysis program (which he discusses in the book), which I think is a powerful way to identify imbalances in your body/mind/spirit that need attention. Doc understands quantum physics, has a deeply personal walk with the Lord, and he knows how to apply those principles to health and the physical realm.

Why is the quantum realm exciting? I think it is the science of how the spirit realm interacts with the physical. I did a voice analysis session with Doc, and it was able to pick up on things I had been working on specifically and gave me many great confirmations. It picked up on physical conditions I already knew about (which is great confirmation). But the test also can pick up on spiritual and emotional issues, which is powerful. I knew I was a seer, but it was confirming and confidence building to hear Doc say, "Wow, you are a seer, aren't you?"

His analysis also revealed some hidden things I hadn't found in my Courts of Heaven court work—like some specific Freemasonry repentance work that needed to be done. I had worked my way through Dr. Horner's book, *Overcoming the False Verdicts of Freemasonry*,[1] removing a lot of the generational curses. Still, Doc was able to pinpoint three levels that showed I needed to go back and work through the repentance on a deeper level to break my bloodlines free. The analysis was so specific, that it pinpointed certain Freemasonry levels that I needed to go back to and work on.

Amazingly, the test was able to see other things, including the percentage that Jesus' image is within me. It also showed me the percentage of the Father's voice within my voice. I want to improve that specific percentage, and Doc was able to explain to me in my appointment with him exactly how to do that.

---

[1] LifeSpring Publishing (2025).

This book helps you apply quantum physics to your health and to understand how it all works on a deeper level. You are going to love it!

Wendy Selvig,
Director, LifeSpring Publishing

Introduction

With this book being the third in my *Unlocking Quantum Series*, I must recommend you read the first book to gain a more complete understanding of how quantum relates to the supernatural. From that foundation I intend to share my thoughts on how quantum can enhance our health. When I say health, I am referring to the health of our entire being. Never has there been a time when including our health in the Kingdom viewpoint has been more important. More than helping us remove filters and static (trauma, mindsets, blockages), our entire being is designed to be a gate for Heaven to move through us. We are the Father's boots on the ground.

In this book I intend to cover everything I know at present as it relates to those things that work against our health. This will include nutrition, water (liquids), diet, contrary mindsets, trauma trapped in organs, trauma in the soul, and more. It is not just the spirit and soul that we must conquer in order to be one with Him. Our body must be part of the picture so that we present our full selves to Him. If we can accomplish this, we will not only walk under an open heaven; we will be a gate for Heaven to flow through.

Being one with Jesus is more than a metaphor. It involves studying, making choices, and learning to walk in a level of "presence" that affects every bit of our three-part being. It is like we are the Rich man to whom Jesus said, "Give all that you have and follow me." That man went away sad because he had been controlling his religious life to his satisfaction. Now, however, he knew he would be asked to do things outside his religious comfort zone. He knew that when the Lord invited us to be one with Him, he (the rich man) would no longer be in control.

If you have read my first two books, you know the quantum grid is the universal operating system that is in place as a result of God speaking order to creation. It is the scientific explanation for how all things are held together and kept by His Word. Armed with this knowledge, a person must decide if they want to be *reactive or proactive* in how they address their earthly assignment. For example, do you accept misbehavior at work, in relationships, and in your health?

Yes, health, because the human body needs to be brought under the Kingdom plan (blueprint) that God has for each one of us. The process of bringing our person into a full Kingdom dynamic makes it easier to pray for others when God has done something powerful in us first.

The first two books in the *Unlocking Quantum Series* have laid out foundational principles that should give us enough information to interact with the quantum grid and, therefore, build our faith. Working on ourselves and practicing the 5-step process for interacting with quantum should give us plenty of practice while we establish our confidence level. Let's remember that the source that we tap into is paramount for our success. To be clear, there is a bad stream and a good stream to draw our inspiration from. The latter has a very narrow access point and is maintained through *relationship*. The former masquerades as individual autonomy while putting that person into an ever-increasing spiral of bondage.

Just like our Savior exemplified, we stay out of error and pride as we only do what we see Father do. Building out the intuitive mind is a critical skill we must develop to stay on the narrow path of carrying out Father's orders. Take a look at John 5:19:

So Jesus answered them by saying, I assure you, most solemnly I tell you, the Son is able to do nothing of Himself (of His own accord); but He is able to do only what He sees the Father doing, for whatever the Father does is what the Son does in the same way [in His turn].

Working on our physical body may be one of the most difficult things we are called to do. The reason that the body is so difficult to work with is because of its direct attachment to 3-D reality. 3-D reality acts as a dampening factor that fights against the light and living water that we should be exuding as ambassadors of Heaven. In short 3-D reality loves to mess with our head with the goal of reducing the level of Kingdom flow we are able to release.

When we accept Jesus as Lord and Savior, our spirit is regenerated and our soul sanctified. Then there is our physical body, which is our footprint on planet Earth. It is against the body that our enemy has formulated plans to keep us distracted on many fronts.

The concept of unlocking quantum health is more than just feeling better. It is allowing the way God wants to move through us to be fully unencumbered. And this even down to the smallest detail of DNA, cellular structure, and our tissue being able to release His incredible light into the darkness of Earth. This darkness is in many forms; however, the most profound is how 3-D tries to limit the wonders of God's love and majesty that He desires for His creation.

The physical body is the last frontier that, when conquered, is the vessel that Father uses to release His design and presence into creation around us. To give us encouragement for our assignment, God went to the trouble of putting His name within our DNA, proving we belong to Him. Let's see how we can make our physical body an equal partner with our spirit as we pursue Kingdom fulfillment.

Chapter 1
Quantum Review

The *quantum realm* refers to the unseen world that affects what we can see, such as molecules, atoms, and protons. It also connects to spiritual principles that go beyond what we can perceive with our physical eyes. The influence of quantum energy comes from beyond the normal world we experience, operating outside of time and space.

A key idea about quantum is that it is part of the Creator's design. When He said, "Let there be," He set everything in motion. It is through His presence, His Word, and His power that everything holds together and stays in order. To understand this better, take a look at Genesis 1 for yourself:

> [1]*In the beginning God (prepared, formed, fashioned, and) created the heavens and the earth.*

² The earth was without form and an empty waste, and darkness was upon the face of the very great deep. The Spirit of God was moving (hovering, brooding) over the face of the waters.

³ And God said, Let there be light; and there was light.

⁴ And God saw that the light was good (suitable, pleasant) and He approved it; and God separated the light from the darkness.

⁵ And God called the light Day, and the darkness He called Night. And there was evening, and there was morning, one day.

⁶ And God said, Let there be a firmament [the expanse of the sky] in the midst of the waters, and let it separate the waters [below] from the waters [above].

⁷ And God made the firmament [the expanse] and separated the waters which were under the expanse from the waters which were above the expanse. And it was so.

⁸ And God called the firmament Heavens. And there was evening, and there was morning, a second day.

⁹ And God said, Let the waters under the heavens be collected into one place [of standing], and let the dry land appear. And it was so.

¹⁰ God called the dry land Earth, and the accumulated waters He called Seas. And God saw that this was good (fitting, admirable) and He approved it.

¹¹ And God said, Let the earth put forth [tender] vegetation: plants yielding seed and fruit trees yielding fruit whose seed is in itself, each according to its kind, upon the earth. And it was so.

¹² The earth brought forth vegetation: plants yielding seed according to their own kinds and trees bearing fruit in which was their seed, each according to its kind. And God saw that it was good (suitable, admirable) and He approved it.

¹³ And there was evening, and there was morning, a third day.

¹⁴ And God said, Let there be lights in the expanse of the heavens to separate the day from the night, and let them be signs and tokens [of God's provident care], and [to mark] seasons, days, and years,

¹⁵ And let them be lights in the expanse of the sky to give light upon the earth. And it was so.

¹⁶ And God made the two great lights—the greater light (the sun) to rule the day and the lesser light (the moon) to rule the night. He also made the stars.

¹⁷ And God set them in the expanse of the heavens to give light upon the earth,

¹⁸ To rule over the day and over the night, and to separate the light from the darkness. And God saw that it was good (fitting, pleasant) and He approved it.

¹⁹ And there was evening, and there was morning, a fourth day.

²⁰ And God said, Let the waters bring forth abundantly and swarm with living creatures, and let birds fly over the earth in the open expanse of the heavens.

²¹ God created the great sea monsters and every living creature that moves, which the waters brought forth abundantly, according to their kinds, and every winged bird according to its kind. And God saw that it was good (suitable, admirable) and He approved it.

²² And God blessed them, saying, Be fruitful, multiply, and fill the waters in the seas, and let the fowl multiply in the earth.

²³ And there was evening, and there was morning, a fifth day.

²⁴ And God said, Let the earth bring forth living creatures according to their kinds: livestock, creeping

things, and [wild] beasts of the earth according to their kinds. And it was so.

²⁵ And God made the [wild] beasts of the earth according to their kinds, and domestic animals according to their kinds, and everything that creeps upon the earth according to its kind. And God saw that it was good (fitting, pleasant) and He approved it.

²⁶ God said, Let Us [Father, Son, and Holy Spirit] make mankind in Our image, after Our likeness, and let them have complete authority over the fish of the sea, the birds of the air, the [tame] beasts, and over all of the earth, and over everything that creeps upon the earth.

²⁷ So God created man in His own image, in the image and likeness of God He created him; male and female He created them.

²⁸ And God blessed them and said to them, Be fruitful, multiply, and fill the earth, and subdue it [using all its vast resources in the service of God and man]; and have dominion over the fish of the sea, the birds of the air, and over every living creature that moves upon the earth.

²⁹ And God said, See, I have given you every plant yielding seed that is on the face of all the land and every tree with seed in its fruit; you shall have them for food.

³⁰ And to all the animals on the earth and to every bird of the air and to everything that creeps on the ground— to everything in which there is the breath of life—I have given every green plant for food. And it was so.

³¹ And God saw everything that He had made, and behold, it was very good (suitable, pleasant) and He approved it completely. And there was evening, and there was morning, a sixth day.

The fall of man changed the Earth and introduced a new system that disrupted its natural order. In essence, the fall diminished creation's ability to remain in resonant harmony with its Creator. Now, creation seems to be struggling, almost as if it's on life support, waiting to be restored to its original beauty and purpose. This is where we come in.

Bringing higher-order designs into our 3-D Earth is part of the mission given to humanity. This was Adam and Eve's purpose, and it's still ours today. Add to this the possibility that what went on in ages past and the pre-flood era may be "energetically" bleeding over into our present age, adding to the depth of what we are called to reset. We have a lot on our plate, so we need to be fully able and fully equipped to get the job done.

Quantum terms like bilocation, quantum entanglement, and wave-particle duality all illustrate what Albert Einstein famously referred to as "spooky action at a distance." The purpose of my *Unlocking Quantum Series* is to help people recognize that what God has established is far more than an abstract or elusive spirituality drifting aimlessly. Rather than relying on mere chance, our Creator has put everything in order so that His children have a verifiable platform and culture to operate from.

Our adversary understands how this system works. So, how does he spread darkness, knowing he has a limited number of fallen angels and resources? He knows that if he can influence just one generation to begin engaging with him, that corrupt mindset will be passed down to future generations (as seen in 2 Timothy 3:1-3). Once the enemy has a person's ear, then he can superimpose his system in the place of the One we were created to operate in. Part of his plan is to throw us off our game by misdirecting our focus. He does this by keeping us busy with nonessential pursuits and multiple forms of spiritual enlightenment that masquerade as Christianity, mysticism, and self-improvement, just as 2 Timothy 3:1-3 suggests will happen:

> *¹ But understand this, that in the last days will come (set in) perilous times of great stress and trouble [hard to deal with and hard to bear].*
>
> *² For people will be lovers of self and [utterly] self-centered, lovers of money and aroused by an inordinate [greedy] desire for wealth, proud and arrogant and contemptuous boasters. They will be abusive (blasphemous, scoffing), disobedient to parents, ungrateful, unholy and profane.*
>
> *³ [They will be] without natural [human] affection (callous and inhuman), relentless (admitting of no truce or appeasement); [they will be] slanderers (false accusers, troublemakers), intemperate and loose in morals and conduct, uncontrolled and fierce, haters of good.*

All true humans are created in the image of God (Genesis 1:27). That image contains a great deal of authority even if that person has yet to be restored to relationship with their Creator. The enemy wants that authority aligned with his plans and system. Basically, they are vampires that try to drain every drop of spiritual authority out of us. They also know our words can enable the creative side of the quantum grid. The enemy wants a culture in place, so we activate that grid for destructive purposes by sending ripples through the grid with our words (knowingly or unknowingly). Culture is what carries captivity or freedom throughout the generations. The question each of us must answer is which culture we wish to be entangled with. It's one or the other, as a mixture really doesn't work!

Chapter 2
The Health of Our Spirit

What I am about to share will be controversial to some. There are multiple reasons it could be; however, the main reason is that we have very limited information about the human race beyond six to seven thousand years ago. All that seems to be in the archaeological record prior to the six-plus thousand years wasn't us. My best guess is that the pre-Adamic record on Earth was the result of life before the introduction of mankind to planet Earth. When mankind was introduced to Earth, it was to begin the process of cleaning up the mess.

The lack of evidence has left theological minds to assume that we came into being the moment that heavenly spark was implanted in our mother's womb. I'm not so sure this is the case. Jeremiah 1:5 tells us that He knew us before we were formed in the womb. There are only two ways to interpret this verse. Either Father had us in His mind before we were born, or we existed as spirits before we came here. I believe the latter. John 17:24 is another verse that hints at our preexisting earthly assignment. I am well aware of the ramifications of this viewpoint; however, we must be mindful that part of the enemy's plan is to throw us off our game. If we were preexistent then we need to know the possibility exists that we could bring "spirit baggage" with us.

This is the only thing that explains the anomalies in my testing that seem to indicate spirit wounds that are not of earthly origin. I'm sure you understand how troubling it can be to find issues that defy normal explanations. Thankfully, God's Word does give us insight as long as it isn't taken as metaphorical information only. It is totally up to you which thread of thought you choose to believe. I only ask that you are open to an expanded revelation.

Jeremiah 1:5 says:

Before I formed you in the womb I knew [and] approved of you [as My chosen instrument], and before you were born I separated and set you apart, consecrating you; [and] I appointed you as a prophet to the nations.

And John 17:24 states:

Father, I desire that they also whom You have entrusted to Me [as Your gift to Me] may be with Me where I am, so that they may see My glory, which You have given Me [Your love gift to Me]; for You loved Me before the foundation of the world.

When we seek to build a case based on evidence, we must consider both the direct and indirect evidence. Scripture is the direct evidence, while things like near-death experiences (NDEs), personal encounters, and individual memories are indirect. The latter carries less weight than the first; however, we must be careful not to dismiss these out of hand. I saw a video of a three-year-old boy shaking his brother, who was about a year and a half old, asking him if he still remembered Heaven. Also, a man named Roy Mills has a book on Amazon where he shares his testimony of asking God to allow him to remember his time in Heaven before he came to Earth. His story is fascinating.

Add to this multiple testimonies of people visiting Heaven as the result of NDEs or by invitation who asked the Father what those spirits were that were flying in and out of Him. Father's answer was that these were the spirits of humans yet to be born on Earth. Perhaps we need to be reminded that in court cases, the testimony of multiple people telling the same story is enough to result in a conviction or acquittal.

Our preexistence is important for two reasons. The first is that we may have to consider "spirit baggage" that needs to be addressed before we can freely execute our assignment. The second is that part of our assignment could be to undo chaos that has been bleeding over from past ages. So, what could have seeped over from the past ages?

We know there was a great war in Heaven. In the human experience, it has barely been 125 years since we have had motorized vehicles and just 40 years since we have had access to computers. This makes it difficult for us to imagine the level of technology that could have existed in ages past, right up to the time Noah entered the ark. Read this account of Revelation 12:7-10:

> *[7] Then war broke out in heaven; Michael and his angels went forth to battle with the dragon, and the dragon and his angels fought.*
>
> *[8] But they were defeated, and there was no room found for them in heaven any longer.*
>
> *[9] And the huge dragon was cast down and out—that age-old serpent, who is called the Devil and Satan, he who is the seducer (deceiver) of all humanity the world over; he was forced out and down to the earth, and his angels were flung out along with him.*

> *¹⁰ Then I heard a strong (loud) voice in heaven, saying, Now it has come—the salvation and the power and the kingdom (the dominion, the reign) of our God, and the power (the sovereignty, the authority) of His Christ (the Messiah); for the accuser of our brethren, he who keeps bringing before our God charges against them day and night, has been cast out!*

If we go back to previous ages, it is quite likely that you and I functioned in some way as a part of the "greater picture" on behalf of the Father. As such, we could have been friends with angels and other beings before the great rebellion. (Our distant ancestors were likely affected by the Genesis 6 rebellion as well). Is it not impossible that some of our friends took part in the great rebellion? If they did, then it could have left us with a wound. It hurts now when someone betrays us, so it likely would have hurt us then. We could have been lied to and even fooled to a certain extent. This would really hurt.

So, I bring this to your attention because we need to be aware that a wounded spirit will diminish our Kingdom's effectiveness. Fortunately, the human voice carries the imprint of this possibility, and I can test for it. While I may not be able to tell you the exact nature of the wound, I can tell how many, and with that information, a person can <u>repent</u> and ask the Father for <u>healing.</u>

It helps when we learn to call our spirit forward on a daily basis. This puts our spirit in charge and establishes us as a spirit-led (our spirit) person who then can walk knowingly in God's presence for the day. Our spirit, being the leader, also sends a message to our soul and body to pay attention and to be cooperative.

Chapter 3
The Health of the Soul

In 2023, I asked the Lord why some wellness clients didn't respond as well as others to the nutritional protocols I can test for. He gave me an open vision of the human soul and revealed that some people have trauma running in the background. He stated this was soul-based and tied into our emotional grid. As a result, He gave me what I call the Holo-Psyche assessment format.

The Lord went on to reveal that even after we have granted forgiveness and had deliverance (if needed), the energetic value of that trauma could still run in the background. I got a picture of what this energy looks like. It looks like balls of plasma that are about the size of a tennis ball. These balls of plasma can anchor in the soul as well as in the organs of our body. It appears that these plasma balls can interact with the quantum grid. This may explain why they seem to take on a life of their own. Once in place this programming needs to stir up trouble so they can feed off of emotional disturbances in order to stay firmly in place. This may also reveal a hidden component of addiction that needs to be addressed.

I am thankful that the Lord gave me a four-step process (that I teach in *Unlocking the Quantum Kingdom*) for excising the trauma. His wish is for us to be free on every level (body, soul, and spirit).

Genesis 2:7-9 says that God breathed into Adam, and he became a living soul. I have stated in all my books that we are NOT restored to the image of Adam when we are born from above. Rather, we are a totally new creation (2 Corinthians 5:17). Romans 8:29 says that we are conformed to the image of His Son, which is a higher design than Adam. This is the epitome of turning lemons into lemonade! Take a look at these three scriptures:

1. **Genesis 2:7-9**

   [7] Then the Lord God formed man from the dust of the ground and breathed into his nostrils the breath or spirit of life, and man became a living being.

⁸ And the Lord God planted a garden toward the east, in Eden [delight]; and there He put the man whom He had formed (framed, constituted).

⁹ And out of the ground the Lord God made to grow every tree that is pleasant to the sight or to be desired— good (suitable, pleasant) for food; the tree of life also in the center of the garden, and the tree of the knowledge of [the difference between] good and evil and blessing and calamity.

2. 2 Corinthians 5:17

Therefore if any person is [ingrafted] in Christ (the Messiah) he is a new creation (a new creature altogether); the old [previous moral and spiritual condition] has passed away. Behold, the fresh and new has come!

3. Romans 8: 29

For those whom He foreknew [of whom He was aware and loved beforehand], He also destined from the beginning [foreordaining them] to be molded into the image of His Son [and share inwardly His likeness], that He might become the firstborn among many brethren.

God first breathed into Adam, and the second Adam breathes into us when we are baptized in the Holy Spirit, and we get fire to boot (John 20:22). This second breath builds upon the first and enables the fullness of this higher design. The "fire" part of the baptism in the Holy Spirit serves to reignite our soul. This is necessary to renew clarity to the role our soul plays in our daily walk.

And having said this, He breathed on them and said to them, Receive the Holy Spirit! (John 20:22)

As 3 John 1:2-4 says, we are to be in health and prosper even as our soul prospers. We can rightfully deduct that the human soul needs to be free and fully functional for us to do all that God has put on our plate.

[2] Beloved, I pray that you may prosper in every way and [that your body] may keep well, even as [I know] your soul keeps well and prospers.

[3] In fact, I greatly rejoiced when [some of] the brethren from time to time arrived and spoke [so highly] of the sincerity and fidelity of your life, as indeed you do live in the Truth [the whole Gospel presents].

[4] I have no greater joy than this, to hear that my [spiritual] children are living their lives in the Truth. (3 John 1:2-4)

Chapter 4
The Health of the Mind

Perhaps you are wondering why we are addressing the mind before the body. The reason is that the mind plays a key role in processing what comes first through our spirit, then through our soul, and then to the body. As I shared in my book *Unlocking Quantum Relationships*,[2] the mind is limited to the frequency base that we have allowed to make up our reality. We are born into an environment and culture that reinforces the logical mind. However, in order to interface with the spirit realm, we need to establish an *intuitive* mind.

When a person has any spirit or soul issues, it is likely that those issues have become a part of that person's reality. It is helpful if these are addressed early on. Then, we can

---

[2] Scroll Publishers (2025).

move on to mindsets that come from culture, family environment, education, and personal choices. Here is where God's Word is vital as we replace inferior belief platforms with those of the highest design.

> *Study and be eager and do your utmost to present yourself to God approved (tested by trial), a workman who has no cause to be ashamed, correctly analyzing and accurately dividing [rightly handling and skillfully teaching] the Word of Truth. (2 Timothy 2:15)*

We must be totally honest as we look through areas of our being. We must seek a vision of God's plan for our lives and then compare that to our present state. This includes the way we think about and address life. The perspective we have chosen to operate from will affect our words when we express our opinions and emotions. If our reality is narrow and only draws from what we can see, then we will have a limited ability to interact with the quantum grid. And when we do interact it will most likely be with negative results. Honesty requires that we see anything outside of God's plan as something that needs to be replaced with His higher design.

Love says it has never been about us. It is about God's plan, and that plan includes expanding our reality so that we can release life in our words to people and the atmosphere around us (Romans 8:19). Love moves us to be proactive and less reactive. When we are proactive, we are looking and listening for ways to make everything around us better. Being reactive means we are allowing life and circumstances to dictate to us. Here is Romans 8:19:

For [even the whole] creation [all nature] waits eagerly for the children of God to be revealed.

As I have repeatedly stated in my books, we cut our teeth on fixing ourselves. It is in this process that we show God we mean business. It is in this process that we build the maturity needed to address things that are well beyond what we could naturally handle. We are completely new creations because we are born from above. This means the supernatural is natural to us, and we need to act like it. The presence of God should be oozing out of every fiber of our being.

To clearly perceive what our spirit sees, we must develop our intuitive mind. The mind constructs inner imagery based on the frequencies that shape our reality. For this inner vision to be accurate and actionable, our minds need to be properly aligned and programmed. This transformation happens through time spent in worship, studying God's Word, and dwelling in His presence. I cannot stress enough the importance of anchoring our minds in the Mind of Christ as Colossians 3:2 says:

And set your minds and keep them set on what is above (the higher things), not on the things that are on the earth.

So, I ask you, are you focused on the things above or things below?

Chapter 5
Doing More Cleanup

In case you are already on overload, I stated that I was going to cover everything I knew. Yes, there is more to consider, namely spiritual legalities. When addressing quantum health, we have to ponder why some folks just need a precise nutritional plan while others still struggle.

DNA

While "spirit baggage and soul traumas" are a revelation to many people we still need to look at DNA that could be altered as well. These alterations would come from generational sin and agreements. For those who dismiss generational sin and agreements, be reminded we still suffer generational amnesia due to the fall in Eden. Therefore, it is not farfetched to think about the possibility that generational sin exists. Technically it is the behavior patterns of sin that are programmed into human DNA that are passed down.

These patterns can be inherited both as behavioral tendencies and genetic predispositions. Even modern science supports this idea. In one study, researchers exposed a group of mice to trauma while simultaneously releasing the scent of roses. They observed that, for at least four generations, the offspring of these mice exhibited panic whenever they smelled rose, even without experiencing the original trauma. This demonstrates how deeply ingrained certain responses can become, offering valuable insight for us to consider.

So, at the very least, behavior patterns and propensities are passed from generation to generation. In John 14:30-31, Jesus says Satan has nothing in Him. This should be our standard and our goal, knowing we are secure in Christ Jesus. Put the logical mind aside and step into the intuitive mind and listen to the inner voice of the Holy Spirit as He will reveal where you stand generationally. Lingering issues indicate a legal document in the spirit realm that stands as an outstanding warrant against you. The same could be said for agreements or vows made by our ancestors. This passage in John has Jesus discussing how Satan has nothing legal he can claim on Him. May we be able to say the same! Here is John 14:30-31:

> *³⁰ I will not talk with you much more, for the prince (evil genius, ruler) of the world is coming. And he has no claim on Me. [He has nothing in common with Me; there is nothing in Me that belongs to him, and he has no power over Me.]*
>
> *³¹ But [Satan is coming and] I do as the Father has commanded Me, so that the world may know (be convinced) that I love the Father and that I do only what the Father has instructed Me to do. [I act in full agreement with His orders.] Rise, let us go away from here.*

To resolve this a person needs to do a heavenly court case. I recommend going to Dr. Ron Horner's website and purchasing his book on the Courts of Heaven. His ministry is also available to do an advocacy session to assist you in discovering issues and also help bring resolution. This can lead to levels of freedom that would have seemed impossible not long ago. Charge your DNA with faith!

Sensory Overload

A functional issue that requires our attention is that of *sensory overload*. We all have TVs, cell phones, and computers, and we are bombarded with news 24/7. This can lead to sensory overload. I recently watched a video about a woman whose ministry focus was in Africa. She went on to share how the children under her care regularly have heavenly visitations and wonderful dreams. When asked why the children in America are deficient in this area, she said it was sensory overload and cultural norms. The African kids do normal things. They play outside, have family time, and read their bibles. Could sensory overload be the source of inner conflict that moves so many in Western culture to seek counseling? Satan's plan keeps us busy.

Union

Another area that needs to be addressed is that of union—union within our person and in relationship with our Creator. While I addressed these in depth in my book *Moving Toward Sonship*,[3] it is worth pointing out that we are here on assignment. Because we are we need to be at the top of our

---

[3] LifeSpring Publishing (2023).

game. Being on top of our game is not possible with the casual level of intimacy (inner picture of Jesus) the majority of believers walk in. The purpose of being born from above is far more than getting a ticket to Heaven and then being careful not to lose that ticket.

Once we realize that we have direct access to Father's heart we can then see ourselves as He sees us. Standing in His love changes us like nothing else can. And once that love has captured us, we can then pass it on to others. In quantum, we send magnificent ripples of power throughout the dimensions as we demonstrate acts of kindness and love to others. Unselfish acts have effects far beyond one person. Those acts can stop the enemy in his tracks and move the recipient to a better mindset. If we are happy then it is so much easier to pass it on to others. Also, because frequencies don't lie, the spirit realm knows if we do something because we must or because we choose to act out of love.

When Satan goes around like a roaring lion seeking whom he may devour, what exactly is he looking for? I propose he can see what spirit a person is operating in and if that spirit is deficient, he pounces on that person. Consider 1 Peter 5:8:

Be well balanced (temperate, sober of mind), be vigilant and cautious at all times; for that enemy of

> *yours, the devil, roams around like a lion roaring [in fierce hunger], seeking someone to seize upon and devour.*

Why does love cover a multitude of sins? (1 Peter 4:8) As tedious as all this "working out our salvation with fear and trembling" seems to be (Psalm 2:11, Philippians 2:12), if we allow love to be the foundation of all that we do, that love will extinguish selfish behavior. Remember, we have choices. I choose to walk in love no matter how hard it may be. God doesn't need me to be the behavioral or doctrinal purity fact-checker of others. He does need me to be His boots on the ground example of His love. I believe hell is real and forever once a person is there. A person who experiences God's love is more likely to keep serving Him as opposed to a person accepting Christ out of fear alone. Consider these verses:

> *Above all things have intense and unfailing love for one another, for love covers a multitude of sins [forgives and disregards the offenses of others]. (1 Peter 4:8)*

> *Serve the Lord with reverent awe and worshipful fear; rejoice and be in high spirits with trembling [lest you displease Him]. (Psalm 2:11)*

> *Therefore, my dear ones, as you have always obeyed [my suggestions], so now, not only [with the*

enthusiasm you would show] in my presence but much more because I am absent, work out (cultivate, carry out to the goal, and fully complete) your own salvation with reverence and awe and trembling (self-distrust, with serious caution, tenderness of conscience, watchfulness against temptation, timidly shrinking from whatever might offend God and discredit the name of Christ). (Philippians 2:12)

A Revelation of Quantum Truth

The focus of this book is the health of our entire being. I will share more practical things about the body in a bit. However, we need to know that our body holds the memory of sin, emotional trauma, and physical trauma in our organs, nervous systems, and endocrine systems.

Sin leaves an imprint because we have formed an agreement with something outside of God's plan for our lives. The moment we are born from above, we are freed from the penalty of our sin; however, we still have a memory of what we did. That memory has an energy value, and that energy value must be addressed. The same goes for any physical and emotional trauma we have experienced.

These memories and energy values serve as markers that are visible in the spirit realm. They leave us open to spiritual attacks that play against our minds as we are in the process of renewing our minds. All of these need to be identified and eliminated. We need to know that the frequencies that the energy values put out serve as gateways to any entities that have been assigned to us. They use these gateways to hijack our thought process, hoping we can be moved to commit sin. The goal is to erode the moral base we received at our new birth. If we do sin, we are likely to speak words that empower our enemy even further.

On the physical side, if our organs or endocrine systems are in bondage to sin or trauma, these systems are put on overload. Those systems are being called to do double duty, which is why we show up with all kinds of symptoms first, and then they eventually turn into disease. This strategy describes a slow yet calculated burnout formulated by our enemy, which few are even aware exists.

What science terms the subconscious mind is really the way our spirit works through our central and autonomic nervous systems. Basic physics tells us that any electrical system must stay within its designed capacity, or there will be a shortage somewhere. This is why breaker switches or fuses are a part of the electrical systems in our homes. We are designed to have our spirit move along the same wiring as the electrical impulses of the autonomic and central nervous systems. If there is rogue energy in these systems caused by trauma then our soul reduces how profoundly our spirit is able to work through those same systems. Remember, the soul can operate as a protective gatekeeper.

Later in the book I list all the things that are on the tests I use to identify the areas that these traumas may be affecting.

Chapter 6
More to Think About

The human heart is the point of convergence of all three personal realms (body, soul, spirit) according to Hebrews 4:12. Each personal realm has its own frequency base that it operates from. The heart is the starting point of the five-step process I lay out in my book *Unlocking the Quantum Kingdom*. The mind needs to have its reality base (frequencies) expanded in order to effectively process the picture the heart sends to it. Many of us need to speak to the eyes of our heart so our heart and eyes are fully connected to the Father's heart realm. We can expand both our hearts and minds by spending time in the Father's heart (presence) and by speaking God's Word out loud as we read. We can expect increased clarity and power as we make this a part of our daily routine. Have a look at Hebrews 4:12:

> *For the Word that God speaks is alive and full of power [making it active, operative, energizing, and effective]; it is sharper than any two-edged sword, penetrating to the dividing line of the breath of life (soul) and [the immortal] spirit, and of joints and marrow [of the deepest parts of our nature], exposing and sifting and analyzing and judging the very thoughts and purposes of the heart. (Hebrews 4:12)*

Science tells us that the heart has memory, so it should be no surprise that the heart holds the image of who we really are. There is no fooling the spirit realm in what we hold. While the fall of man reduced the heart's visual spectrum, we need to know that Jesus fully restored it. All we need to do is activate it and practice seeing from our hearts. The day that we have our personal life review we are less likely to be judged on our accomplishments and more likely to be judged on how well we loved. Don't be afraid to ask for a heart upgrade. Psalm 51:10-12 is just such a request:

> [10] *Create in me a clean heart, O God, and renew a right, persevering, and steadfast spirit within me.*
>
> [11] *Cast me not away from Your presence and take not Your Holy Spirit from me.*
>
> [12] *Restore to me the joy of Your salvation and uphold me with a willing spirit.*

I recommend putting on special worship music in the background and practicing opening the eyes of your heart. Specifically, try to be more aware of pictures that may come across the viewing screen in the imagination. Most people will see in greyscale at first so do not be afraid to ask God for a color upgrade with the colors of Heaven. The best place to start is to see ourselves the way God sees us. Practice often!

I recently had the privilege of hearing Dr. Ron Horner teaching about reclaiming our crowns. It is obvious we are given crowns, or we would not be able to lay them at Jesus' feet as the elders do here in Revelation 4:9-11:

> *⁹ And whenever the living creatures offer glory and honor and thanksgiving to Him Who sits on the throne, Who lives forever and ever (through the eternities of the eternities),*
>
> *¹⁰ The twenty-four elders (the members of the heavenly Sanhedrin) fall prostrate before Him Who is sitting on the throne, and they worship Him Who lives forever and ever; and they throw down their crowns before the throne, crying out,*
>
> *¹¹ Worthy are You, our Lord and God, to receive the glory and the honor and dominion, for You created all things; by Your will they were [brought into being] and were created.*

The simple way to know if we have lost a crown is that we are no longer able to do spiritual things as we once did. The solution is to identify, repent, pick the crown back up, let Jesus cleanse it and pick it up to walk in it again. This is a little-known yet very important part of our walk.

Another thing we absolutely must adjust to is living out of our past. A great many new believers rejoice at what the Lord has delivered them from. At some point, that needs to fade into the background, and our testimony should be drawn from the new creation we have become. As we break away from any victim mentality, our focus should be on Kingdom exploits and encouraging others to do the same. He set us free from the past, so if a cycle of your past issues is still playing in the background, you need to shut it down. We have free will and many of us are more than able to stop any such cycles. If you aren't able then be honest, you need help. Reach out to those who are skilled in this area.

I encourage you to remember that power can't land if it's all about us. Neither can results be expected if it's all about us.

Chapter 7
The Human Body

I have often wondered why the human body wears down the way it does. I have contemplated where viruses, bacterial infections, and parasites came from. I find it hard to believe they were an issue to Adam and Eve before their transgression.

No doubt, the environment that embodies the Tree of the Knowledge of Good and Evil *(Bad Tree)* has something to do with this. I can only come up with two possibilities that are related. The first is that the enemy developed viruses, bacterial infections, and parasites to wear us down. Perhaps they served a different function before the fall, and that function was altered to become the pathogens that plague us today. The second is that they are simply the byproduct of the fall. Either way we have to deal with these because they are the root of nearly all diseases known to mankind. Exceptions would be radioactivity and manmade pathogens.

I will not go into depth at this time; however, we also need to be aware of what we eat, how much we eat, and why we eat as we do. The same goes for what we take in the form of liquids. *Food and drink should empower us, not comfort us.*

The good news is that my testing protocols can find nutritional deficiencies and also identify parasitical, viral and bacterial issues. I use the information I get from the electromagnetic impulses of the body that tell your story when I do my testing. They have been found to be extremely accurate, and I have often found issues before they showed up in medical testing and in the testing of other alternative modalities. I am able to recommend specific nutritional protocols to cover each need.

We do know that we are of the Father's design, and He is able to heal us on every level we seek Him. Most people lack a personal plan, and that is what I specialize in. The body is important because we are God's boots on the ground. We need a strong energy field that is able to release His light without being diminished in any way. A healthy body is, therefore, necessary to accomplish this. For some, it is easier, and for some, it takes longer, yet all we need is the resolve and the will to see it through.

I watch Sid Roth's program quite a bit. Several of his guests have had personal visitations from Jesus. Regularly the Lord Jesus tells them to tell people that healing has already been done for them. That means we just need to walk healing out in faith. No doubt the Lord doesn't mind if a person gets a "faith boost" from those who operate in greater faith than the person needing healing.

I am reminded that the unsaved need healing, too. What a way to demonstrate God's love toward the unsaved by demonstrating healing. This is a part of our Kingdom demonstration and a part of the "greater things than these." So, believers need to accept what is already done while we demonstrate God's love by releasing healing to the unsaved.

Speak healing scriptures out loud to the body. This will engage the co-creative magneto-electric part of our assignment. Regularly engage the fire, glory, presence, light, and living water of God. Also, practice the five-step sequence mentioned in my book *Unlocking the Quantum Kingdom*. Practice builds proficiency.

One thing I am sure of is that the more light we contain the harder it is for the enemy to wear us down physically.

Chapter 8
Our Emotions

Our emotional stability plays a big role in how our physical body operates. Just as research has shown that bad programming in the soul can affect us, so too can emotions that run like bad programming in the background. Some Bible teachers mistakenly attribute mind, will, and emotions to the human soul only. We have found that each realm (body, soul, spirit) has its own set of mind, will, and emotions. This means that the body has its way of storing memory, as do our soul and spirit.

It is known by modern science that the entire digestive system has an equal amount of memory cells, as does the brain. They call this the "gut-brain connection." The implication is that our digestive system has its memory. Of late others have discovered that our organs are able to retain the memory of certain traumas.

I recently watched a documentary about a person who received a heart transplant from a person who was brutally murdered. The person who received the transplant was able to identify the murderer because of the memory that remained in the victim's heart, and that memory was accepted by the court as being valid.

I like to reference the works of Henry Wright because he shows how diseases find their root in our emotional spectrum.

For example:

- Anger—tension in neck and shoulders, general headaches and migraines, high blood pressure, skin conditions.
- Fear—fast heartbeats and palpitations, panic attacks, digestive issues and insomnia.
- Guilt—low self-esteem, physical depletion, mid-lower back pain, IBS.
- Shame—upper body tension, Jaw pain, constipation, poor posture.
- Grief—shortness of breath, chest pain, fatigue, low energy, stomach pain, nausea.

Situations faced as a child...according to Dr. Natalia (last name withheld):

- Emotions dismissed by others = back pain.
- Suppressed feelings = anxiety disorder.
- Being overlooked and unimportant = control issues.
- Absentee parents = survival mode.
- Not being good enough = perfectionist.
- You were the peacekeeper = migraines.
- Only feeling safe by pleasing others = autoimmune.
- Shamed for being vulnerable = feeling unsafe with intimacy.
- You were the caregiver = chronic stress or depression.

While this list is not comprehensive, it gives you an idea of how important it is to address things that we have been taught to dismiss or just push down inside. To be fair, we just did what we thought was right at the time. Some people do cope better than others.

The thing about the quantum field is that one percent of quantum responds to any human, and the enemy is aware of this. This means that one percent responds to both the good and the bad. The reason that it does is that it is a part of God's overall system that He put into place when He spoke all things into existence. How this relates to you and me is that when we experience trauma, that trauma draws a bit of creative substance when it forms. It then goes on to create a quantum memory that finds its home somewhere in our body. Now, that would be bad enough; however, once that memory is in place, the memory seems to reach out to quantum in order to get stronger. You could even say the memory takes on a life of its own. In the beginning, the person being affected knows something isn't right. So they go to the doctor, and the doctor runs all kinds of tests and rarely finds anything. If that person goes back often enough, the doctor is likely to prescribe antidepressants. This could lead to a cycle of prescription drug dependence until a disease eventually shows up. This shows you the power of emotional energy. It also shows how modern medicine has no way to evaluate what trauma and trapped emotions can do to the body.

Oh wait, it gets better. The same thing can happen in our digestive system. Emotions like anger, anxiety, sadness, abuse, and rejection can all settle in our digestive system. Once an emotion settles in, the result could be any number of symptoms. From the gut, syndromes like IBS, anxiety attacks, malabsorption syndrome and GERD may actually start as the result of a trauma. Once a diagnosis is made, the doctor may prescribe drugs, and most drugs have side effects. This can often lead to more prescription meds and a never-ending cycle, all to keep us busy chasing better health and reducing our time to grow in Kingdom.

I hope you are beginning to see that humanity must be pretty special and be a threat to the enemy's plans for him to go through all the trouble to come up with such a complex plan to render us ineffective. This is why it is vital to spend some time daily in our place of rest, which is the Father's heart, and while there, we can engage His emotional realm to get a better picture of what ours should look like. His light heals on so many levels.

Fortunately, there is good news. Everything our Savior did for us includes the emotional realm, along with any symptoms that may result. Also, I have developed a new test that shows how traumas and emotions can affect the organs and endocrine system. The test rates each system from one to ten. Anything less than ten is an issue and then I am able to identify the corresponding emotion. The four-part protocol that works to release trapped energy in the soul also works for trapped emotions in the body.

Chapter 9
Hormones and More

Hormones are stress and regulatory substances designed to keep our organs synced to the quantum field. Our nervous system is regulatory and gives our spirit a physical expression.

Our soul is the seat of *power* for our intent and emotions. The soul also filters the frequencies given off from the intention of others. It also provides the quantum energy our voice needs to release Heaven's higher designs. When our organs are in good shape, they work with our cellular structure to broadcast frequencies that expand our energy field so we can interact with quantum at a high level. Our spirit synchronizes with the frequencies of Heaven that are then passed down the chain of command.

The enemy hates it when he sees a person whose body works well, so he loves to put people into stressful situations.

If he can accomplish this then the resulting toll it takes on our wellbeing causes irregularities in hormonal production. Stress can result in too much or too little hormonal production. This can cause all kinds of symptoms. And back to the doctor we go, and the cycle starts all over again. Dysfunctional hormones mean our organs have trouble synchronizing with the quantum grid. This is the goal of our enemy.

Soaking in the presence of meaningful worship music can be a big help to soothe all the chaos that leads to energetic hormonal responses. This is why getting sensory overload under control is so important.

My testing modality can pinpoint hormonal imbalances. Fortunately, I can suggest nutrition that will help a person build up their hormonal reserves.

Chapter 10
DNA

DNA plays a key role in how God uses us to speak His will into the Earth. Science recognizes DNA's role in how we develop physically. Unfortunately, science normally doesn't look into the spiritual link that DNA has. DNA's spiritual link is that it is an antenna that magnifies what our mind feeds into it. DNA broadcasts to empower our cells so that we may expand our energy field. Expanding our energy field is how we are able to interact with the quantum grid and bring things from outside of space and time into 3-D Earth reality.

I recently watched a video that explained that the way DNA is assembled in the body bears the signature of God. His name is literally written into our DNA. Obviously, this means no question about Who made us and Who we should belong to. This builds our faith.

In my book *Moving Toward Sonship*, I explained how we need to invite the spirit of Purity to walk through our DNA with us. Purity has the authority to repair our DNA and remove both physical and spiritual anomalies. For those folks who engage the supernatural regularly, it is normal to ask Heaven for assistance. For those who are not familiar with engaging Heaven, then simply do it by faith. Being stretched is part of the Kingdom process, so give it a shot. I have received many testimonies about the changes that have taken place in those who have asked the spirit of Purity for assistance.

DNA is in the 5-step process of expanding our energy field to interact with the quantum field. That process is as follows: an idea moves from the heart to the mind, and then the mind sends the frequencies of the idea to our DNA. Our DNA then communicates with our cells that light us up like a Christmas tree. At that point, we start to become more wave than matter. Being more wave than matter creates a link to resources that are outside of space and time. Understanding this process breaks down things we have done by faith into more scientific terms. I am personally comforted by knowing how things work whenever possible.

So, I encourage you to link up with the spirit of Purity and let Purity lead you to heal your DNA physically and generationally. Ask Purity to restore your generations (mantels) within you and also to help format your DNA with all Father wants you to walk in. This would include gifts, signs, wonders and miracles! My response is, "Ok, devil, you want to play games? Now we see what God can do within me!"

Chapter 11
My Medallions

This is an entirely new field that came to my attention in October of 2023. All I was attempting to do was make a medallion that reduced electromagnetic signals from Wi-Fi and TV. One day, I was assembling materials to make several of these medallions, and the Lord asked me this question, "What would happen if you put gemstones in your base formula?" I answered that I didn't know but sure hoped that He would tell me.

It turns out that when specific gemstones are put in acrylic resin, they create a unified frequency that promotes moments of **electromagnetic clarity in our personal energy field.** This is important because we are bombarded with chaotic energy from both the natural and spiritual realms. When the bad energy is neutralized, we are able to hear with greater clarity what our spirit knows. These are great aids as we seek to bring greater clarity into our walk as a believer.

Let me be clear: there is a bit of opposition in the body of Christ about crystals and gemstones, which I believe stems from a lack of understanding. I have been amazed at how a person reads an article and suddenly they are an expert on the New Age. Many who disparage the use of gemstones and crystals still use their cell phones, which use crystals. Many wear jewelry without giving it a second thought. Do they contain gemstones? Oops!

Keep in mind that I know how to do very sophisticated testing of the body's energy field (naturally and spiritually). I have tested people before and after wearing medallions, and the results are shocking to the positive. Many of us "old timers" remember crystal radio sets that used clear quartz crystals to tune radio stations. I guess that makes those old radios evil as well. People in the New Age movement and occult use certain crystals to boost their intention. Do we have another case of Christians throwing the baby out with the bath water? Knowing our source is critical in order to walk in Kingdom purity.

Like many things on Earth, they can be used for good and evil. The naysayers would do well to remember that each time they turn on a computer, that computer can be used for good or evil, just like gemstones and crystals. By the way, the High Priest of Israel wore an Ephod made of gemstones to get answers from Heaven. Also, gemstones are mentioned throughout the Bible as being building materials there.

In the appendix of my book *Unlocking the Quantum Kingdom* I have a testimony from a person who had a heavenly visitation that spoke all about the medallions I put together. At present, I have 18 different variations of medallions that are related to topics of engagement. Be sure to visit my website for more information.

Chapter 12
Diet, Exercise, and Personal Discipline

Earlier I stated that food should empower us, not be a reward to us. My expertise is in clinical nutrition which is the application of nutraceuticals to improve wellness. I am not a dietary expert; however, after doing wellness evaluations for thirty years, I have learned a few things. If you need expert dietary advice, be sure to ask a dietitian.

Years ago, I came across a diet plan by Dr. Peter D'Adamo called the "Eat for Your Type Diet." It seems that we break down foods differently based on our blood type. The plans laid out in his book have proved to be very helpful. Also helpful is the knowledge of combining foods so that they will digest more easily and not fight against each other while digesting. I do the carnivore diet a couple of times a year as a way to detox and help my body heal.

Exercise

Exercise can always be a blessing if done correctly. Since I am no longer interested in showing a six-pack at the beach, I focus on stretches and squats that keep my muscles toned. Walking is a great benefit to the body if a person is able. Recently, I saw a video made in Great Britain by a doctor who took twenty old people who had many health issues. He had them build up to the point where they could walk for thirty minutes a day for at least five days a week. The results were that many of their symptoms disappeared, and each reduced the number of medications they were on.

Diet

Scripture says our body is the temple of the Holy Spirit (1 Corinthians 6:19). I am here to tell you that this has more than spiritual connotations. I'll never forget an evangelist who told a joke about his wife putting him on a liquid diet. He said the protein shake tasted pretty good with a half-gallon of ice cream mixed into it. Sadly, he weighed every bit of 400 pounds. He did get some good laughs. Consider 1 Corinthians 6:19:

> *Do you not know that your body is the temple (the very sanctuary) of the Holy Spirit Who lives within you,*

Whom you have received [as a Gift] from God? You are not your own.

I have a very serious question to ask. Is God obligated to heal us if we neglect our responsibility to eat properly and show personal discipline with our lifestyle? I get those who have underlying medical issues have a harder time, yet how could eating better, exercising properly, and showing personal discipline by getting proper sleep hurt us?

When I look at beach pictures from the 1970s versus the way people look today, I am shocked. As people blessed with free will, we are free to make choices. Most of the foods we eat have horrible additives in them. Many foods are genetically modified, and the water bottles we drink from leach estrogen. As believers, we need to make better choices, and it must be more than talk. An unhealthy lifestyle diminishes the body's ability to release godly frequencies to the creation around us. And that is what this book is all about, putting our body into the best possible place to do Kingdom exploits.

Water

Have you ever thought about why God invented water? Why not something else? We could ask if water has a spiritual significance. Water can be solid, liquid or gas. Is this a type of how the Creator uses His triune design throughout nature? Water flows from His throne. Why does Heaven even need water? This is another matter for Kings to search out. What we do know is that God does nothing without reason or purpose.

Attributes of water:

- Water cleanses and purifies.
- Water acts as a solvent.
- Water hydrates.
- Water can heal.
- Water connects us to all other forms of life (that need water).
- Water has memory.
- Still water reflects an image.
- Water can be programmed (structured).
- Water responds to prayer.
- Water has sentience.
- Water has crystalline properties.
- Water conducts electricity.

YouTube is full of videos that show people speaking to water and praying over it. The water is in a glass container and then frozen. When viewed under a microscope water shows pleasant or troubling designs. I saw a video of a lady who asked water what her name was, and the initials of her first and last names were visible under a microscope. When water is prayed over, it shows beautiful designs. When disharmonic sounds are played near water it shows scary designs.

Could the role of water be to remind all creation and creatures how they need to depend on Him? Consider these verses in Romans 1:18-20:

> [18] *For God's [holy] wrath and indignation are revealed from heaven against all ungodliness and unrighteousness of men, who in their wickedness repress and hinder the truth and make it inoperative.*
>
> [19] *For that which is known about God is evident to them and made plain in their inner consciousness, because God [Himself] has shown it to them.*
>
> [20] *For ever since the creation of the world His invisible nature and attributes, that is, His eternal power and divinity, have been made intelligible and clearly discernible in and through the things that have been made (His handiworks). So [men] are without excuse [altogether without any defense or justification].*

Have you ever thought about why our water is fluoridated? Science tells us that fluoride calcifies the pineal gland. We need an operational pineal gland to help promote hormonal functions. The same gland is known to help us with intuition and the perception of things beyond the physical realm. So, if the pineal gland is calcified, can we process frequencies? This is another part of Satan's plan, to keep us dull.

Water holds things. Tea, coffee, tincture, color, sugar, alcohol, and fluoride, to name a few. If water holds things, then how does what it contains change its ability to conduct electricity? How would some things water could contain lead to poor cellular response? We already know if our cells do not respond properly to messages from our DNA then we have a hard time expanding our energy field to interact with quantum. It sounds like a gain of function from the enemy's camp as we mindlessly play along.

It is all about the song we carry. We are designed to be tuned by Heaven 24/7. We have a song within us that is supposed to bring all things around us to a higher and restored purpose. That was the norm for all creation before the great cosmic rebellion. And this is a part of our current assignment which we are restored to. If what we take in is polluted, then there would be little doubt the effectiveness of that song will be diminished. And this is true for nearly every aspect of our life.

I believe 85% of all illnesses could be avoided if we drank enough water and prayed over it. I structure my water with a terahertz device. It must be water! I'm not sure Diet Coke can be programmed to benefit us.

Minerals

We live in a time when the vegetables we eat and the ground it is grown in have lost their voice. That voice was enabled by vital minerals that were once in the ground. It is well known in alternative circles that minerals (vitamins, too) that are sourced from the ground that does have minerals in it, help people thrive.

We need minerals to promote electrical conductivity throughout the systems of the body. These are the same systems that give our spirit the ability to express itself within our body. Could this "dumbing down" of our nutrition have been done by design? It does make you wonder.

Chapter 13
Nutritional Testing

Over thirty years ago, I learned to do an advanced form of muscle testing called Contact Reflex Analysis (CRA). I became good friends with the doctor who discovered CRA, Dr. D.A. Versendaal. CRA allows the practitioner to test the meridians of the body for energetic hot spots. These hot spots indicate nutritional deficiencies.

The first test I do is a complete CRA workup. I find *nutritional deficiencies* and make corresponding supplemental recommendations. CRA is also excellent at spotting root problems that traditional doctors seem to be uninterested in addressing. I get it because their focus is to manage disease. It's hard to get repeat business if you cure people. God bless the increasing number of doctors who are waking up and moving to a wellness platform.

The goal of all wellness practitioners is to help the body restore its energy reserves. More energy almost always translates to better health. What I have learned over the past thirty years is that not all wellness modalities have the ability to go to the depth that CRA does. So, absent any underlying spiritual issues that are causing an illness, I would recommend CRA as a good place to start if you are seeking an alternative option.

The Spiritual Assessment

My next test is called the *Spiritual Assessment.* Some years ago, I was asked by some folks who were on their Kingdom journey if I could test for certain spiritual attributes. Since I do most of my tests from the frequencies of the human voice, I said I'd give it a try. As it turns out, I can test for spiritual attributes and much more.

Included in the spiritual assessment are the following:

- Union with the Lord.
- Union with our realms (body, soul, spirit).
- Quantum emotional realm.
- Quantum heart realm.
- Your engagement proficiency.
- How well do you see, know, hear, or feel?

- The level of Father's voice in your voice.
- The strength of Jesus' image in you.
- Your DNA viability (normal DNA pulses at 19, which stands for faith).
- Levels of warfare against you.
- The level of God's fire, glory, and light you operate in.
- How well you benefit from communion.
- The percentage of your scroll you have fulfilled.
- The percentage of your scroll that you understand.
- How well you operate in government.
- The number of spirit wounds you carry.

All of these are scored on a scale of 0-10, with 10 being the best. A score of seven or above is a good place to be. Most of these metrics are to let you know how you are doing in your Kingdom pursuit while giving you a baseline to work off of. I recommend a person repeats all the tests every year.

The Holo-psyche Release Assessment

This test is to find traumatic programming that is based on the human soul. It is programming that is located behind nine organs of the body. The energy is like bad programming that is emitted from the soul and can affect the function of our physical organs. The nine organs are:

- Thyroid
- Heart
- Stomach
- Right psoas muscle (not an organ, an energetic gateway)
- Large intestines
- Liver
- Lungs
- Kidneys
- Spleen

Each organ is tied to a specific set of emotions. First, I identify the affected organ and then identify the corresponding emotion(s). There is a four-step deliverance process that is easy to do, and the results have been outstanding. It is not necessary to rate these issues from 0-10.

Negative Spiritual Attachments

These tests are two pages based on the works of Dr. Ron Horner. I rate the strength of the song you have for each of your realms at 0-10 then I move on to various topics. The harmony we release from our person can change the atmosphere in a room and also affect the creation around us. I recently went to our community mailbox where I ran into a lady who was walking her dog. The dog came right up to me and let me pet her. Her owner was shocked because she said her dog normally barks at everyone. Could the dog sense my good energy?

The topics for Negative Spiritual Attachments are:

- Timelines
- Fractures in body, soul, spirit and if any alters exist
- Regions of captivity
- Agreements, of which eight are listed
- Hidden nuptials (marriage contracts in the spirit) eight are listed
- Emotional roots, which four are listed
- Obstacles which eight are listed
- Bonds of iniquity, which six are listed
- And several miscellaneous items

To be set free from these, a Heavenly court case is often needed. I will point out that Dr. Ron Horner's ministry has very anointed advocates who are familiar with these tests and are able to assist you as you address these.

Regions of Bodily captivity

In this test I test every major organ and body system. These include:

- The brain
- The esophagus
- Stomach
- Small intestine
- Large intestine
- Heart
- Liver
- Spleen
- Thyroid
- Lungs
- Kidneys
- The skeletal system
- The pineal gland
- Male and female systems
- The eyes
- The ears
- The nose (smell), which some say has a quantum connection
- Central nervous system
- Autonomic nervous system
- And more

Endocrine Test

This test covers the thirteen endocrine glands which is where the energetic value of our sin seems to settle in. Once an underperforming gland is identified, I test to see which of the seventeen sins of the flesh are present.

What I am looking for here is the function of each category listed. If it is below 10, I test for an emotional tie. The Regions of Bodily Captivity test draws from a list of 38 main emotions that I test to see if any of the twenty-five categories show less than a 10. Once an issue is recognized I advise the client to repent if applicable and grant forgiveness. There are times when a Heavenly court case is necessary to enable a solution. In other situations, the four-step deliverance process I use in the Holo-psyche release assessment will bring what I discover to a satisfactory conclusion. The four-step Holo-psyche sequence works for both the Endocrine system and Regions of Bodily Captivity issues. As far as I know, there is no one else doing a battery of tests that is this comprehensive.

On my website, I divide the nutritional and spiritual tests into two parts. This means a person can choose either or both. Those who choose both get a combination discount.

Five of the six spiritual tests that I do are trauma and emotional based.

At the end of the day, we are participating in a comprehensive story of redemption. That story includes you and me and the creation around us. This is something we should never forget.

Chapter 14
Heavenly Engagements and Heaven's Wellness Clinic

In my book *Moving Toward Sonship*, I lay out what a spiritual engagement is. I will give a synopsis here. Because Jesus lives in us and we are in Him, we are quantumly entangled. For the purpose of heavenly engagements this means we can exchange information, visuals, and revelation at the speed of thought. For example, when we zero in on being in the heavenly throne room because of the entanglement, our spirit is really there, or we get a picture as if we are there. This is how things work outside of space and time (quantum). If we know this and believe it, we can engage in quantum principles and change the world around us.

Unlike unapproved "New Age" practices, we do not astral project. We don't need to because Jesus is the approved gate (He said that He is the gate), and He is the way to do all we need to do. Doing *only what we see the Father do* indicates that we don't just decide to visit Heaven. We ask and wait for permission. Once we have permission, we call our spirit forward and then engage our intuitive mind and wait for the picture (or living video). Now you can see why we need an expanded reality and a new set of frequencies in the mind so that we get a vivid picture of Heaven's reality.

Because the focus of this book is quantum health, let's say we need to go to one of Heaven's health clinics. Those who live in Heaven do not need a clinic; we do. They are there for us. I realize that this sounds fantastic to some. However, we are reminded that the reason that it would seem fantastic is that we have been programmed to think 3-D is the only reality that exists. Kingdom folks have an expanded dimensional reality, so this is a part of that reality.

Once a person is in the clinic, let the people who are there treat you and guide you just like you would at any clinic on Earth. While many of us do this by faith, the more often we are invited to have engagements the more visual they will become to us. Going to a heavenly clinic should become the norm as our walk in Kingdom advances. And who knows, if times get tough on Earth, we may need to visit a heavenly grocery store to get things we need on Earth. Enoch walked right into Heaven so we could do something similar.

Be sure to email me if you have an experience in a Heavenly clinic. I'd love to hear about it.

Chapter 15
The Blood of Jesus

I would be remiss if I didn't mention the greatest weapon we have in our quest for wholeness. What is that weapon? It is the blood of Jesus. Just think, our Savior was slain from the foundation of the Earth. On the surface this seems to be a foundational religious truth only. As we dig deeper, we see that it has deep quantum connections. Revelation 13:8 gives us a peek into this:

> *All the inhabitants of the earth will fall down and worship him, everyone whose name has not been written since the foundation of the world in the Book of Life of the Lamb who has been slain [as a willing sacrifice].*

Quantum operates outside of space and time. The blood of Jesus was shed from the very beginning of all things being outside of space and time. In quantum, time is circular, and different ages seem to intersect in unique ways. There is no doubt that blood releases its sound in all ages, to all peoples, to all things. It is the only acceptable currency to redeem mankind and restore mankind to family and our assignment.

My question from a quantum perspective is, what does that blood actually hold in its design? We do know it is one of two sacraments in Holy Communion. Perhaps we should expand our thinking as we take communion and engage that body and that blood in a more comprehensive way.

The quantum principles of quantum entanglement and non-locality reflect the idea of spiritual union with our Savior. The "blood" symbolizes an incredible connection that transcends space and time. While the articles of communion are symbols, they could be symbols that, when taken in faith and with sincerity, could tie us supernaturally with our Savior at a very deep quantum level. I believe this, as well as other truths, were hidden from our enemy in ages past.

We know the blood cleanses us from all sin and unrighteousness, but does it also unite us with our Savior on a vibrational and frequency level? And if it does, how deeply do we engage with those vibrations and frequencies (presence)? If we did expand our reality and engage at a deeper level, what changes in our being should we expect?

We also know distance is not an issue. Perhaps this is one of the mysteries that should be sought out by kings as Proverbs 25:2 suggests:

> *It is the glory of God to conceal a matter, But the glory of kings is to search out a matter. (Proverbs 25:2)*

While I do not fully agree with our Catholic friends that the sacraments turn into the literal body and blood of our Savior, they may be leaning in the right direction. In quantum terms, the sacraments quantumly link us with our Savior via the quantum principle of quantum entanglement. The Godhead is quantumly linked because they share the same essence. That essence link means they share the same design and attributes. When we take communion, we are invited to identify with our Savior's essence. Not to become Him yet to be like Him. What an invitation and what love. This should grip us to our very core.

Could taking communion be our invitation to participate in the Divine Nature as a family? Scripture says that when a man and a woman come together, they become one. Science knows that every time a man and a woman are intimate, they exchange DNA. No doubt, communion is a spiritual picture of that union where our Savior shares His DNA with us. And how does He do that? With an ever-increasing transfusion of His blood from deep spiritual intimacy.

A natural example of this is eating a meal. Let's say we stop by KFC and pick up a bucket of chicken. As a piece of chicken is being digested, we benefit from the protein, and that protein gives us energy. By partaking in the chicken, we benefit from the chicken; however, we do not become a chicken. While taking communion we are able to gain many benefits from the person of our Savior while not literally becoming Him.

We are adopted, yet this is not a normal adoption (Ephesians 1:5). Communion enables a deep mystery which is that our blood begins to take on the attributes of His. The bread also enables an interconnectedness with His person. In quantum, this is a form of shared duality. To be like Him yet not being Him. The discerning will understand.

In the past little was known of DNA. Today, there is science that proves it. The real question here is: do you want to wait until you die to undergo a deep spiritual transformation, or will you pursue that change *now*?

That blood regenerates our spirit, and it sanctifies our soul. The purity of that blood assures our access to physical healing and opens the door to interconnectedness if we allow the process to play out to completion. That blood covers us like a shield, that blood covers us like a cloak, and that blood can heal us to the uttermost on every possible level. This is quantum health at its best.

Now that you understand that opening up the eyes of your heart will allow you to see into the spirit realm when you have an engagement, the next time you take communion, ask the Lord Jesus if He wants to take you anywhere. Ask Him if He wants to show you anything. And ask Him to synchronize the power of His blood with your person, to pour His DNA into your being.

Building a new reality means being honest about things that really haven't worked in the past. We can continue to take communion honoring our Lord's sacrifice, or we can do that and add to it the expectation that He wants to change us fully into His image here and now.

Chapter 16
Conclusion

So, what have we learned? We are boots-on-the-ground representatives of our Creator. We are His temple, and we have personal responsibilities for our body, soul, and spirit. After we have addressed anything that creates resistance in our person, we are then free to do the greater things than those that our Savior spoke about in John 14:12-17:

> *[12] I assure you, most solemnly I tell you, if anyone steadfastly believes in Me, he will himself be able to do the things that I do; and he will do even greater things than these, because I go to the Father.*
>
> *[13] And I will do [I Myself will grant] whatever you ask in My Name [as presenting all that I Am], so that the Father may be glorified and extolled in (through) the Son.*

[superscript]14 [Yes] I will grant [I Myself will do for you] whatever you shall ask in My Name [as presenting all that I Am].

[superscript]15 If you [really] love Me, you will keep (obey) My commands.

[superscript]16 And I will ask the Father, and He will give you another Comforter (Counselor, Helper, Intercessor, Advocate, Strengthener, and Standby), that He may remain with you forever—

[superscript]17 The Spirit of Truth, Whom the world cannot receive (welcome, take to its heart), because it does not see Him or know and recognize Him. But you know and recognize Him, for He lives with you [constantly] and will be in you.

We have discovered that we can interact with both God's direct presence and the quantum grid, a fundamental part of creation, to fulfill our assignments. To do so, we must expand our understanding beyond the limitations of the 3-D world we are accustomed to. Many have struggled to step into this reality because they lacked a clear strategy to remove the mental filters, distractions, and limiting beliefs that held them back.

As stated in 3 John 1:2-4, our Heavenly Father desires for us to be in health and to prosper, even as our soul prospers.

This applies to every area of our lives. We are people of faith, yet it can be challenging to operate in the fullness of faith if things are running in the background that force us to take one step back for every two we take forward.

> *² Beloved, I pray that you may prosper in every way and [that your body] may keep well, even as [I know] your soul keeps well and prospers.*
>
> *³ In fact, I greatly rejoiced when [some of] the brethren from time to time arrived and spoke [so highly] of the sincerity and fidelity of your life, as indeed you do live in the Truth [the whole Gospel presents].*
>
> *⁴ I have no greater joy than this, to hear that my [spiritual] children are living their lives in the Truth.* (3 John 1:2-4)

I have laid out many possibilities for you to look into. They help identify any unapproved energy that may be affecting your spirit, soul, and body with its many systems. Identifying these helps equip you to move forward with the health of your total being. My hope is that you will be challenged to expand your reality to the point where living in the supernatural is as common as going to Walmart. The day has come for our full attention to be on things above and not below. Consider Romans 8:19:

> *For [even the whole] creation [all nature] waits eagerly for the children of God to be revealed.*

Our quantum connectedness to the Father's heart gives us the hope that we can see, know, hear, feel and demonstrate God's Kingdom as never before. It shouldn't be long before we hear the call of Creation. When you hear that call, run to it!

The real point of all my books is to describe the basics of quantum and how they apply to the supernatural realm we are to walk in as believers. If we won't take the time to expand our reality so we understand the way things really work, then how are we going to have answers for other people when the veil between the dimensions is pulled back? The things I have presented in my books are kindergarten-level material compared to what we may see in our lifetimes.

You and I have a unique opportunity to get a head start in these things. With that head start, we will have tested the basics of quantum and, in the process, position ourselves for God's response to what we are all about to see. When Father decides to send a greater portion our way, that greater portion must have a foundation to set itself upon. This is the time to get our priorities in order. It is a time to get our minds straight and once again see with the eyes of our hearts.

Keep in mind the church as a whole hasn't been straight with us. Because it hasn't, we can't expect them to see the bigger picture that I am referring to here. So, my advice is to learn about the way the greater spirit realm operates (book 1). Learn how to build relationships with God and people (book 2). And engage the very presence of God to become the most holistically balanced believer that you can possibly be (this book).

May God our Father open His heart to you and bless you in your journey.

(All scriptures are from the Amplified Bible)

Appendix A

What you will find on my website is an explanation of all of my medallions and the two categories of tests that I do. The wellness test is $250.00. The spiritually related tests are $350.00. When you combine them, they cost $500.00, which is a savings of $100.00 if purchased separately.

I use PayPal on the site; however, I can take a check as well. If you email me, I will let you know how we can make a check work.

While the site is relatively simple, if you are in doubt, you can always use the donate button. I will be notified of your purchase and email you very quickly and ask you to tell me what your exact order is. This is also true if you order multiple medallions. Just add the prices up and use the donation button. I will ask which specific medallions you would like and verify your mailing address.

Appendix B

Gemstones

Many have contacted me by email with questions about how all the various medallions that I make could help them. Each medallion has a formula. That formula works with our personal energy field to create a frequency field. The frequency field boosts and enhances our energy field.

The energy set is especially valuable for boosting energy. The medallions that were created by the topic are to be worn while engaging God as it will clarify our own field as we are engaging according to the topic.

Keep in mind that the prices are subject to change, so be sure to check my website for the up-to-date prices.

Gemstones as Frequency Boosters

Since the beginning of humanity, mankind has used gemstones as adornments and a sign of wealth, power, and position. Scripture describes how gemstones serve as building materials in Heaven, but could that be their only purpose? Science has discovered that our cells contain crystalline structures, including the pineal gland with its microscopic crystals. Nicola Tesla once noted that crystals exhibit "living being" properties, with potential uses for sending and receiving frequencies.

Most of humanity gets up every morning without pondering how the universe or creation's fabric is constructed. But just as a light switch is assumed to work, few consider the complexities that make it so. For some, the focus shifts from "Why are we here?" to exploring what surrounds us and how it operates.

Scripture reveals that what is seen and unseen was created by God's spoken Word and empowered by His light. Creation is ordered and kept in order by His Word, and light is its power source, being a part of His essence. He is light, and things are and can be made (of) by light. In that light are countless bits of information, much like that which is carried by fiber optic cables. This tells me that creation may not be static but an ongoing process as His light continually engages the foundational substance of creation that He left in place.

In a perfect environment, His light and those allowed to release His light should have an impact on the ongoing process of creation. However, in the distant past, a cataclysmic rebellion affected this process. That rebellion enabled a dark force to dampen what we see as visible creation.

Scripture speaks of creation "crying out" for the sons of God to be revealed so things can be restored to their original order and balance. This restored order would be very different from the autonomic function around us that we have accepted as normal. In other words, everything is currently on autopilot, which dampens everything around us from expressing things that come directly from the Creator's heart as they were designed to do. We may miss much that was designed for us because we accept this "default mode" of darkness as normal.

In these last days, some are satisfied to have their relationship restored with the Creator as they accept His one and only Son, Jesus Christ, as Lord and Savior. There are, however, others who have been drawn deeper into the story of creation and are pressing in such a way that they have been challenged to use their "light" to answer the call of creation for a more complete restoration. To remove the dampening force so that creation can once again sing its song and reflect the way it was originally designed to be.

Many of us have discovered that a person cannot jump from step one in this process to step ten overnight. There are skill levels to be developed, and understanding needs to be acquired. We first work through the inversion of self to enable a more effective release of that inner light. Then, we can start impacting creation around us.

To be successful in this process, we have many resources to draw from, both spiritually and naturally. Because gemstones both send and receive frequencies and are affected by intent and faith, they are a wonderful aid as we seek to address the fullness of scripture and restore what is around us. Gemstones are frequency boosters that can help clarify things as we seek the face of God in the fulfillment of our earthly assignments.

Gemstones help us work past the static and filters of the soul and body as we seek clarity to grasp what our spirit has known all along. Because God is matter, spirit, and quantum, it is quite possible that the quantum link to His heart was lost in the fall. This would have tremendous ramifications.

I see that gemstones are like bicycle training wheels. They are simply physical tools that can help us clarify what our spirit already knows: the more often we engage Heaven, we will be able to see, know, feel, and hear what is being communicated to us. In this case, *familiarity breeds proficiency.*

Earth has its own operational platform with dampened frequency intensity. Heaven also has its own platform with much higher frequencies and the accompanying intentions of the Father's heart. Upgrading our ability to link powerfully with Father's heart is a game changer.

Let's look at how each medallion category can assist us. And don't forget how faith and intent are the energetic spark to power up what each medallion can do.

Medallions

The Energy Daytime and PM Rest & Contemplation Set   **$105.00**

This basic set is ideal for anyone looking to enhance dream clarity and reduce exposure to electromagnetic frequencies (EMFs). While the full impact of EMFs on our bodies and minds is still being researched, we know they can influence us on multiple levels. The Energy Medallion offers protection by blocking up to sixty-five percent of EMFs and includes carefully chosen gemstones to enhance subtle energies, helping you feel more balanced and focused during the day.

To support relaxation, the PM Medallion helps you unwind in the evening while also providing EMF protection.

Note: Be sure to remove the Energy Medallion by early evening, as its energizing properties may otherwise interfere with your sleep.

The Sleep Medallion $105.00

Designed to block up to 85% of EMFs during sleep, this medallion combines specially chosen gemstones that support rest and promote deeper, more restorative sleep.

The Pain Medallion $105.00

While this medallion was designed to ease those wandering aches and pains, it also does an excellent job of changing EMF patterns that cause migraine headaches.

The Weight Assist Medallion $105.00

By converting personal energy and EMF signals into frequencies that enhance cellular function, this medallion supports weight loss when combined with a balanced diet and regular exercise.

The Focus Medallion $105.00

Different from the PM medallion, this one is designed for increased mental focus. Recently I was experiencing brain fog from a sinus infection and asked the Lord if I could make a medallion to help with mental clarity. The result was outstanding.

Engagement Medallions

Quantum Emotional $155.00

This medallion helps us work on our emotional base and how we process stress and past hurts. With it, we can tie into the Father's emotional realm and reformat our own into His image.

Quantum Heart $155.00

This medallion helps us connect directly with Father's heart. This is important because until we see ourselves as He sees us, we will not be able to function in the full scope of Sonship.

Light/Essence/Arche $155.00

This transformative three-part medallion facilitates a profound connection with both your inner light and the Father's light. It enhances engagement with creative essence, empowering you to interact with the creation around you in meaningful ways. Additionally, it allows you to reconnect with your original design from ages past, reinforcing confidence in the unique, wonderfully made nature of your being.

Engaging Holy Fire $155.00

Scripture reveals that God is Light, Love, and Fire—each expressing essential aspects of His nature. Other descriptions we encounter in Scripture help us understand His qualities more fully. Fire, in particular, acts as a profound cleanser. It has the power to purify us on many levels, removing impurities and strengthening what is good. We all need time in an environment where His refining fire can eliminate the dross within us, leaving only what is true and enduring.

Engaging Glory $155.00

We all benefit from a clear vision of God's honor and magnificence. Like all medallions, they serve to elevate our understanding and inspire us to embrace a higher standard of living. Through these symbols, we hope to receive and embody the qualities of His greatness in our own lives.

The Seer Medallion $155.00

Like its namesake, this medallion will help boost frequencies, so we see better in our way of engaging Heaven. It may even boost a person's dream life.

The Breath of Life Medallion $155.00

This medallion is for the more advanced Kingdom seeker where, rather than depending on Earth's physical oxygen as their source of life, that person relies on the Breath of God. While we are still learning exactly what this looks like, there is no doubt that pressing into higher realms for a higher design will serve us well in the future.

The Ephod $155.00

These are the twelve stones worn by the Jewish High Priest (or gemstones with identical frequencies). This is a true governmental medallion focusing on getting answers on governing self, family, job, finances, and our geographical area. It has a lot of energy, so choose wisely when to use it.

The Mazzaroth $205.00

This remarkably high governmental medallion helps us govern from the cosmos, especially the part where our personal story is written. We are still learning the nuances of this medallion, so feedback is always welcome.

The Morningstar $205.00

Like the Mazzaroth, this medallion denotes an even higher Cosmic calling in some ways. According to 2 Peter 1:19, we have an indication that when the greater release of Christ in us takes place (it's a process), there should be an exponential release of our light and His light in the areas of our focus. This is obviously worth looking into.

Immortality $205.00

We are still learning about this; however, we know that immortality is promised in numerous scriptures, not just Heaven. How do we get there? This medallion will undoubtedly help.

I can say that this is so powerful that unless you have your scriptures ready and your focus in place, it may cause headaches or discomfort. It is obviously not for the faint of heart or to be worn as just jewelry.

Engaging 3-D Reality $205.00

While like the essence part of the Light/Essence/ Arche medallion, this medallion is for engaging the fabric of 3-D reality to see what you have been called as a son or daughter to engage and bring to a higher design. This can be on Earth or the near cosmos as it relates to anything that creation is crying out for as long as it is part of God's design.

The Destiny Medallion $255.00

This medallion is what Heaven says; it is the gemstone that will best help you fulfill your scroll and engage your destiny. It takes a voice print to draw from and then many hours of testing the hundreds of gemstones available to choose from to assemble your special medallion. You could say this is the frequency equivalent to the nutritional workups I do.

Doc's Face & Wrinkle Cream $30.00/jar

This blend of healing and essential oils rejuvenates your skin and helps remove the smaller wrinkles while lessening the bigger ones. Many ladies also use this as a base for their makeup.

The cost is $30 per jar, and unless accompanied by a medallion order, they are shipped in sets of two.

. . . .

Also, my books *Moving Toward Sonship, Unlocking the Quantum Kingdom,* and *Unlocking Quantum Relationships* can be ordered from Amazon and Lulu.com.

Website: **docrodich.com**
Email: **doc.rodich@gmail.com**

Description

Unlocking Quantum Health invites you into a deeper understanding of health through the lens of the Kingdom and quantum revelation. As the third book in the *Unlocking Quantum Series*, it builds on foundational truths about how God's design, expressed through the quantum grid, holds all things together—including your spirit, soul, and body.

In this volume, Dr. Rodich explores how nutrition, trauma, mindsets, and the physical body intersect with your divine assignment. More than just achieving wellness, this journey is about becoming a clear, unhindered gate for Heaven to flow through.

When your whole being is aligned with God's blueprint, even your DNA and cellular structure can carry His light into the darkness of Earth. This is not theory—it's a call to bring your physical body into Kingdom partnership, so your presence becomes a vessel of divine healing and transformation.

Step into quantum health and become fully one with Him.

About the Author

Dr. Robert Rodich, author of *Unlocking the Quantum Kingdom* and *Moving Toward Sonship*, is a dedicated scholar of the quantum realm and its profound connections to spiritual growth. With a long-term fascination for how quantum principles can inform and deepen one's understanding of faith, Dr. Rodich's writings invite readers into a journey of exploration that challenges the boundaries of traditional spirituality. This book offers practical insights into how quantum ideas can transform perspectives and lead to personal empowerment and spiritual awakening.

Dr. Rodich shares his life with his wife, Laura, and together, they are blessed with a large family of seven sons and eleven grandchildren. His family has been a continual source of inspiration, encouraging him to explore how science and spirituality intersect to unlock potential within us and our world. Dr. Rodich's work inspires those seeking a deeper connection to the divine through the fascinating lens of the quantum kingdom.

For inquiries, contact him at:
Email: doc.rodich@gmail.com
Website: docrodich.com

Published by:

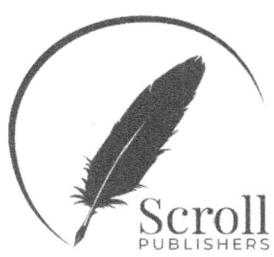

A division of LifeSpring Publishing

www.scrollpublishers.com

Has God spoken to you about writing a book?
Let us help you!